Let's Learn
CANNABIS

An Informational Print
for Children
By A. Chamberlain

Author & Illustrator
Amber Chamberlain

Citations
THC image pg. 4 -
https://en.wikipedia.org/wiki/Tetrahydrocannabinol

CBD image pg. 6 -
https://en.wikipedia.org/wiki/Cannabidiol

Terpene Profile pg. 8 -
https://www.kindpng.com/imgv/imiximh_types-of-odor-causing-ter-penes-in-cannabis-hd/

HerLife HerWrite Publishing Co. LLC
ISBN: 978-1-7349232-9-2

For my daughter, Cadence. The sweetest soul I know..

-Mommy

Let's Learn

CANNABIS

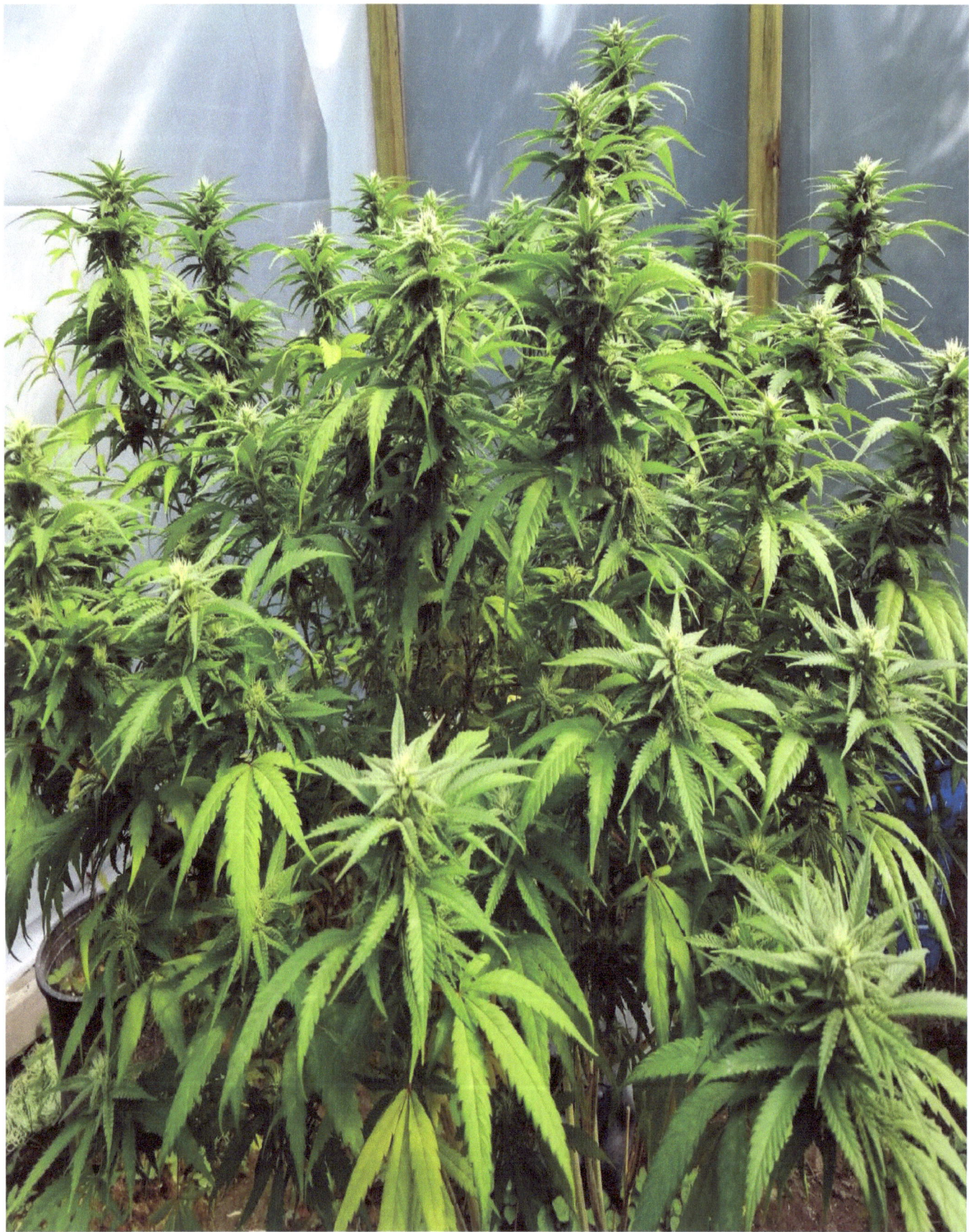

The Cannabis Plant

This is what the plant looks like when it's <u>blooming</u> or flowering. This plant has many uses and helps a lot of people with their pain or sadness.

This plant produces <u>herbs</u> that can be <u>harvested</u> or picked for their uses. It has been growing on the planet for a looooong time!

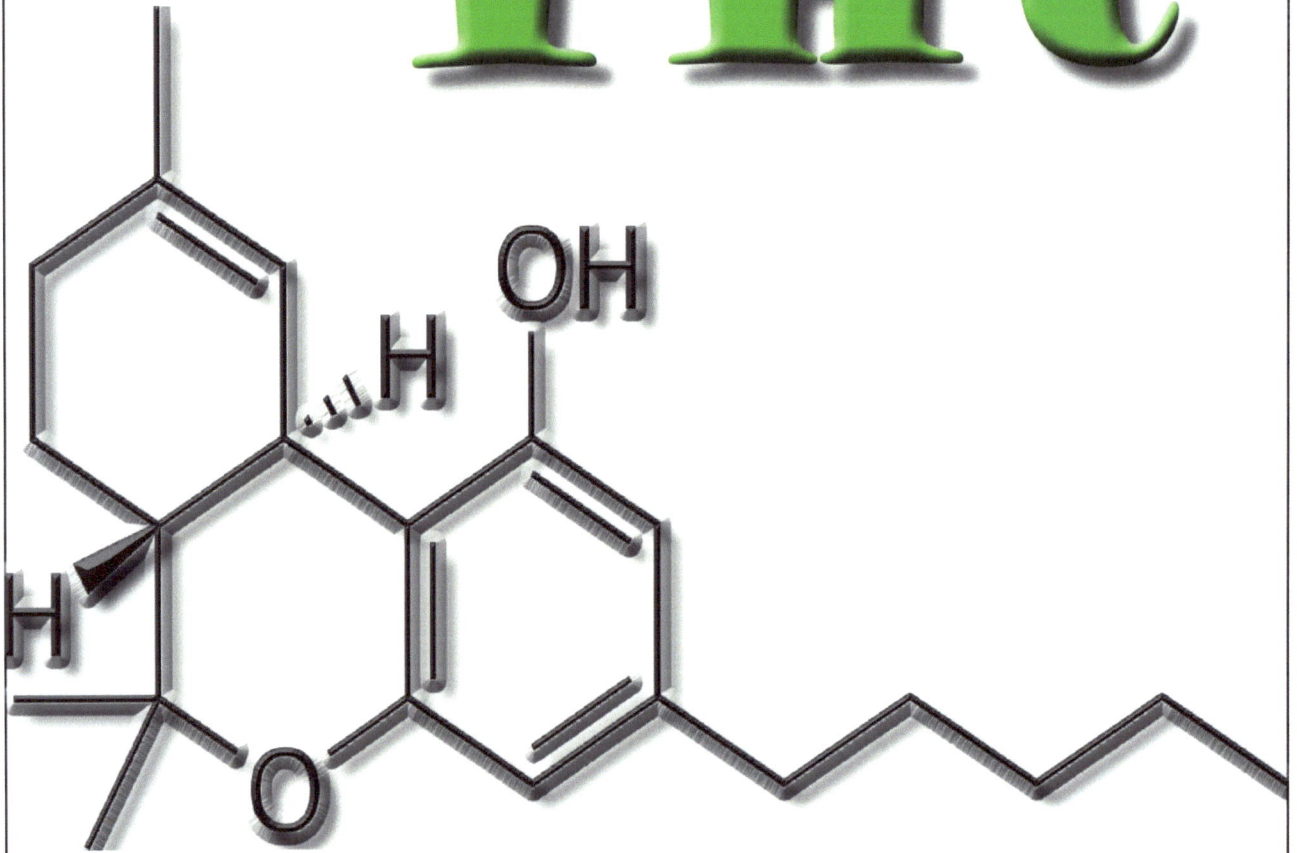

THC – What is it?

THC is also known by its scientific name "Tetrahydrocannabinol."
tet·ra·hy·dro·can·nab·i·nol
/tetre-hīdre-k-nabe-nôl/
Now, thats a BIG word! THC is the most common part of the plant that causes the changes you can feel almost instantly inside your body. It is one of the psychoactive (psy·cho·ac·tive) [sīkō-aktiv] properties.

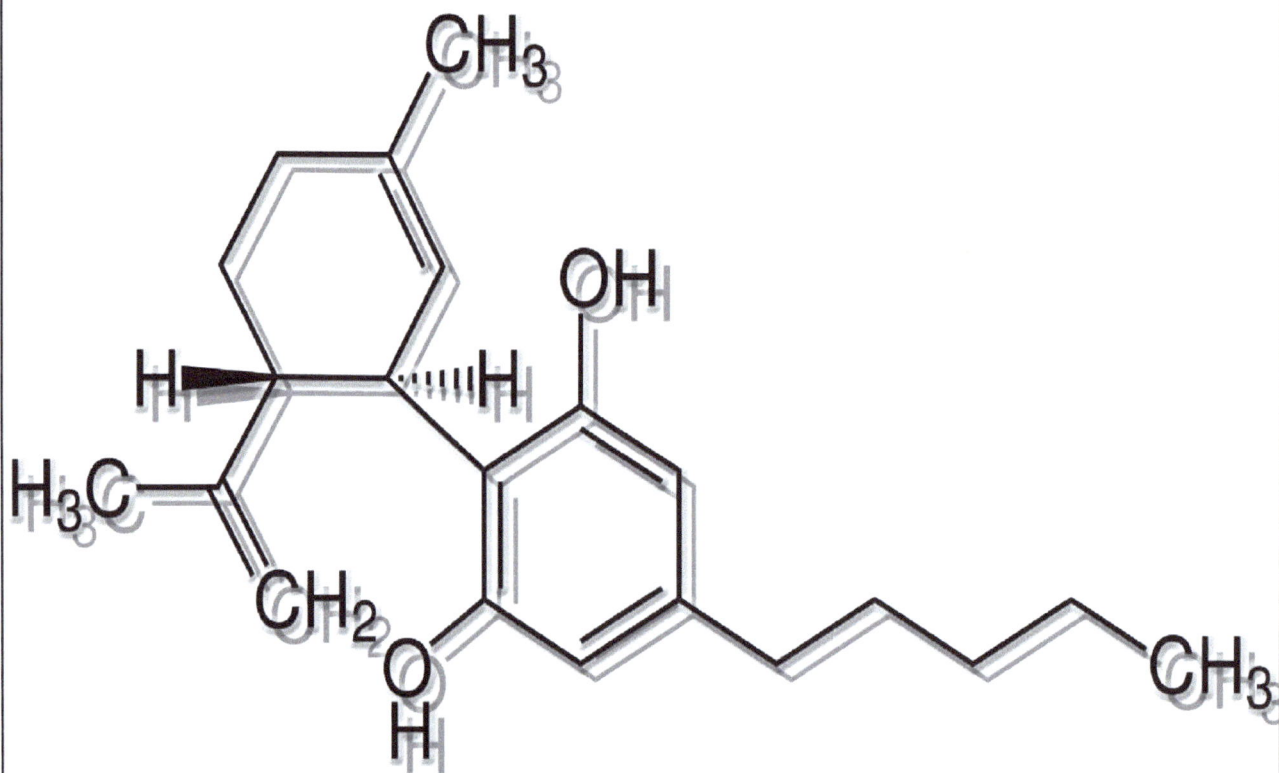

CBD – What is it?

CBD also has another name! Scientists use the name "<u>Cannabidiol</u>." CBD is the other best known <u>cannabinoid</u> of the cannabis plant. CBD is what they call <u>non-psychoactive (psy·cho·ac·tive)</u> <u>[sīkō-aktiv]</u>, meaning you don't feel a change inside your body. People usually use CBD for its calming effects among other benefits.

Here is a list of a few Terpenes found within the cannabis plant.

Terpene	Limonene	Pinene	Myrcene	Linalool	Caryophyllene	Terpinolene	Camphene
Aroma	Citrus, Lemon	Pine, Fir	Musky, Earthy, Cloves	Floral, Lavender	Spices, Black Pepper, Wood	Pine, Herbs	Damp Woods

Terpene	Terpineol	Phellandrene	Carene	Humulene	Pulegone	Sabinene	Geraniol
Aroma	Lilac, Flower Blossoms	Peppermint, Citrus	Sweet, Pungent (Fir)	Hops, Beer	Peppermint	Pine, Orange, Spices	Rose

What are Terpenes?

Terpenes are what give the plant it's smell and flavor. Yes, you are also able to taste the plant. Although, a lot of people don't like that. <u>Terpenes</u> are what your body is attracted to. Some plant <u>strains</u>, or types, you may like but others may not.

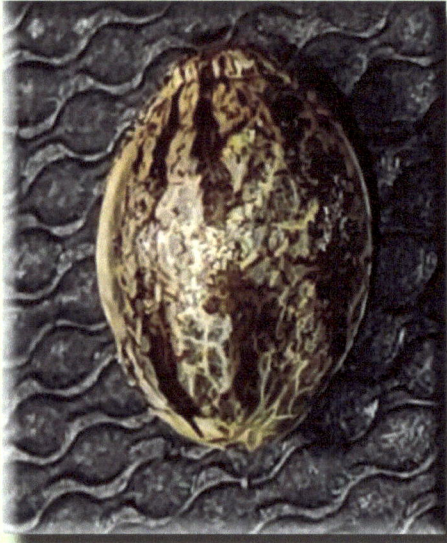

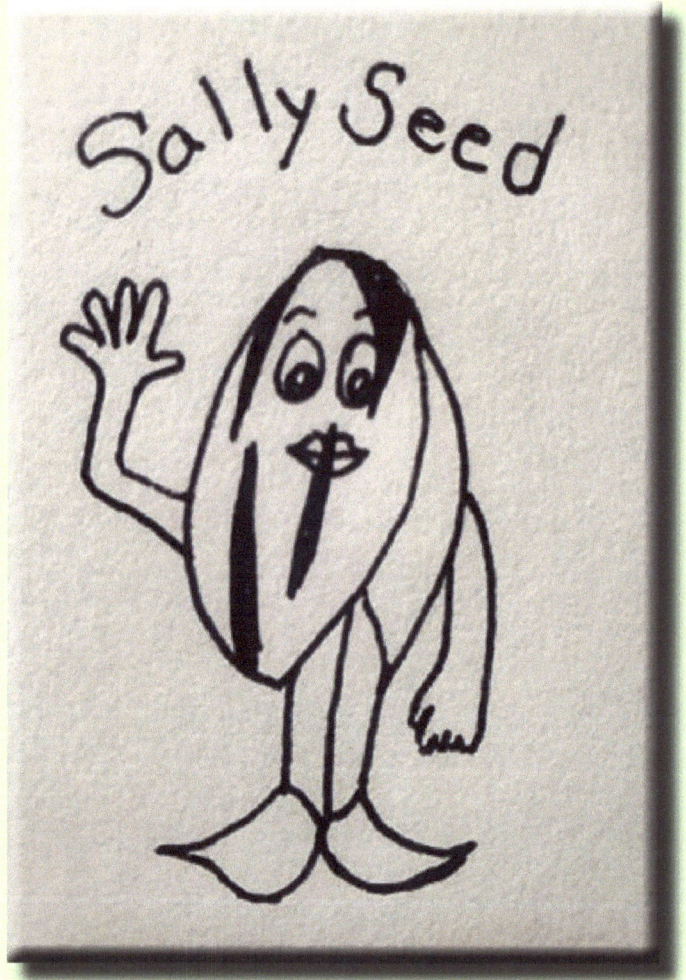

It's Time to Meet our Friends!

To the left, we have Miss Sally Seed.
Without Sally we would have no
plant! Oh no!
Luckily she isn't easily frightened
away.
The seed of the plant is where
everything starts. Once she's ready
(<u>Germinated</u>) she produces a tiny
root to start growing.

Next to Sally is a picture of a real
seed!

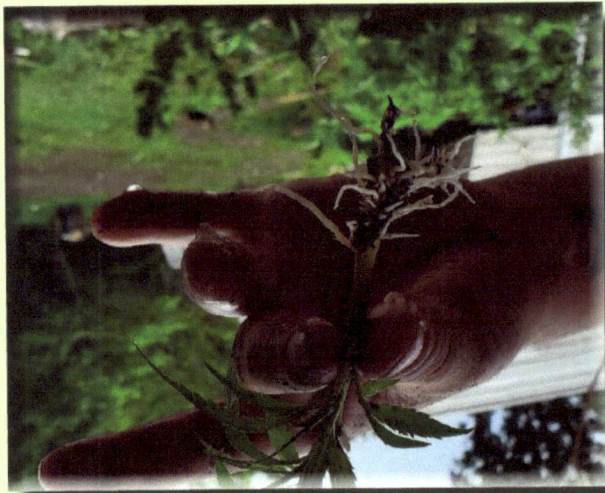

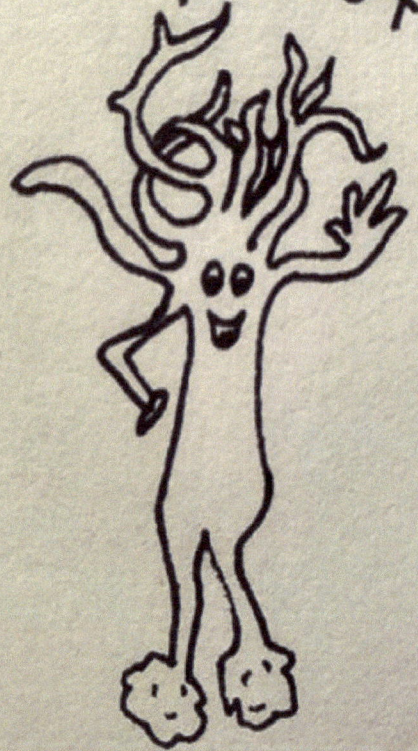

Rodney Root

Meet Rodney Root

When Sally produces her tiny roots Rodney Root comes to life! The root of the plant is where the stem starts. The roots aren't visible when the plant is growing in soil, they like to keep their home dark and damp. The can grow pretty long!

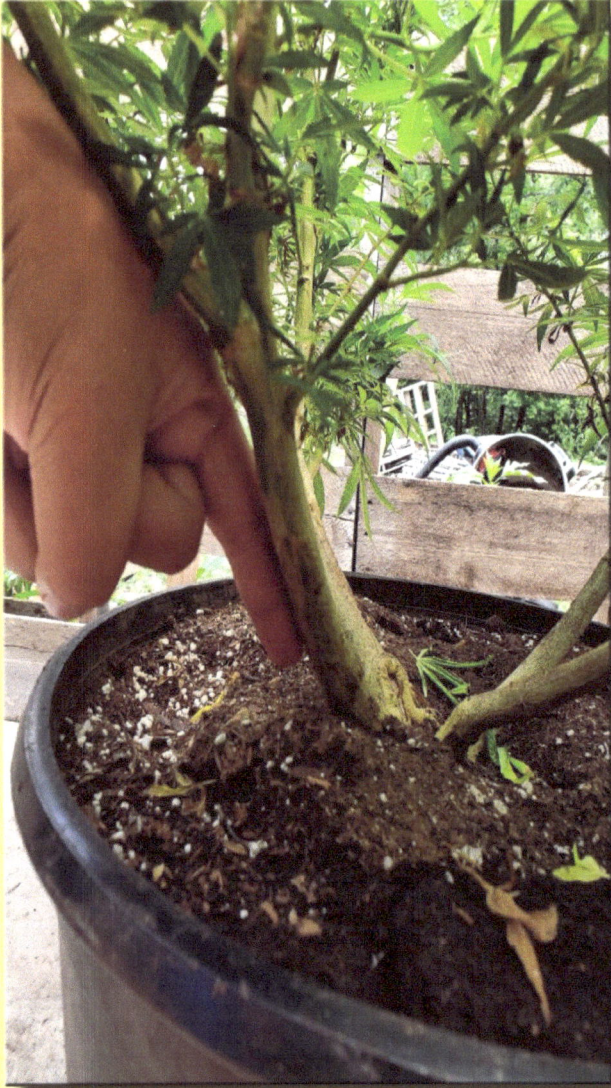

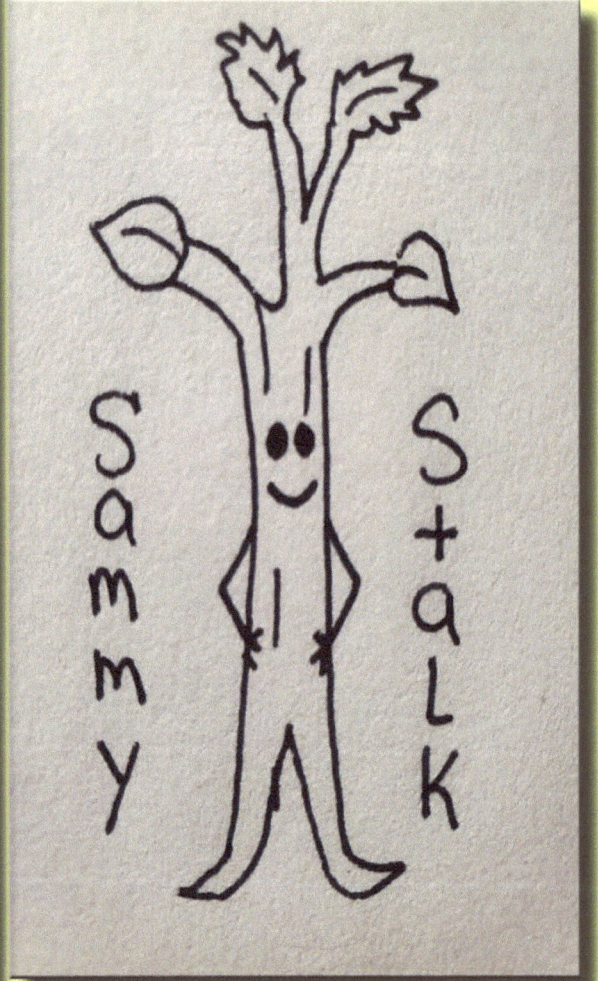

Sammy Stalk

Sammy Stalk

This is Sammy Stalk, Sammy loves to talk! When rodney grows strong enough, Sammy moves in. The stalk grows from the roots which grow from the seed. The stalk is the muscles of the plant that hold everything up! Wouldn't you like to be as strong as Sammy?

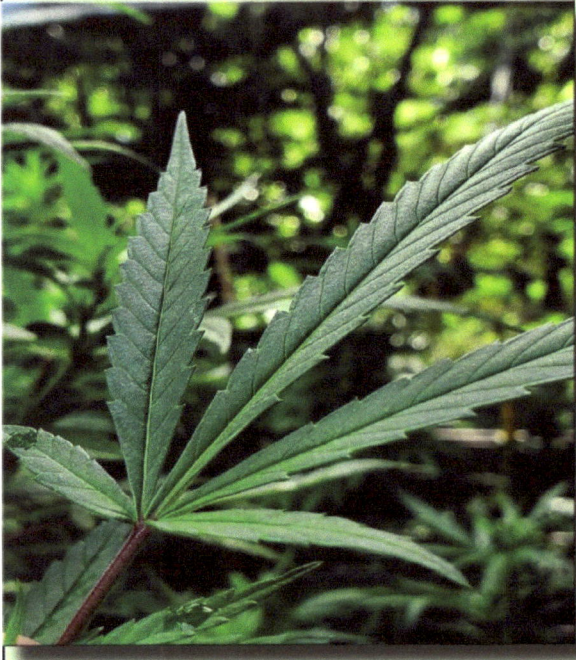

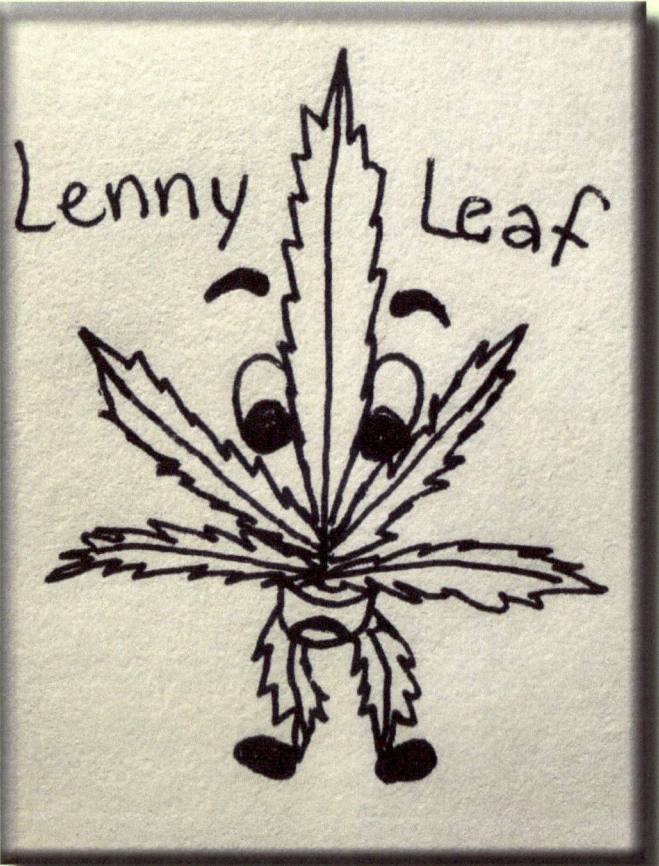

Lenny Leaf

Lenny Leaf

This is Lenny Leaf, once Sammy grows his arms, or branches, Lenny joins the club. The leaf is just as important as the roots.

Leaves soak up all the energy from the lights and certain <u>nutrients</u>, or food to the plants. Leaves can grow as big as your head!

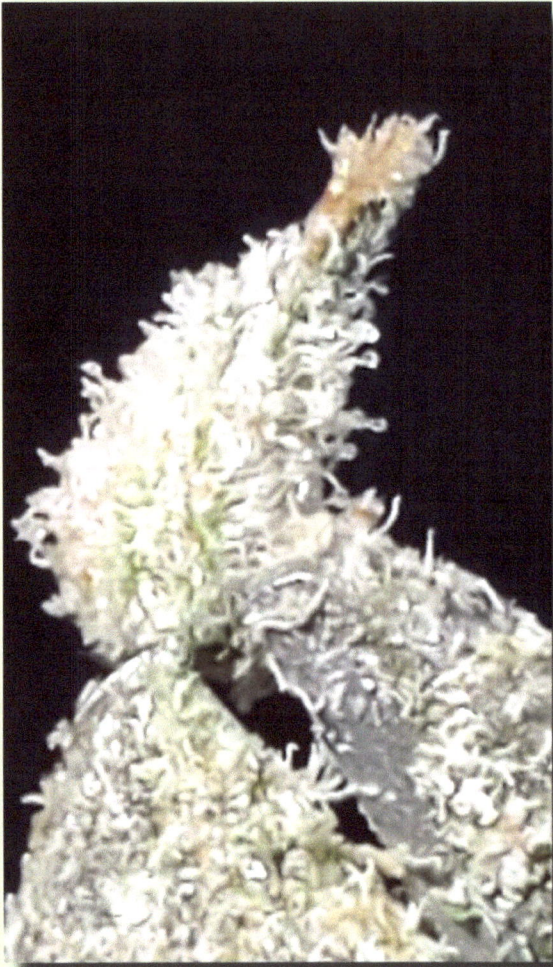
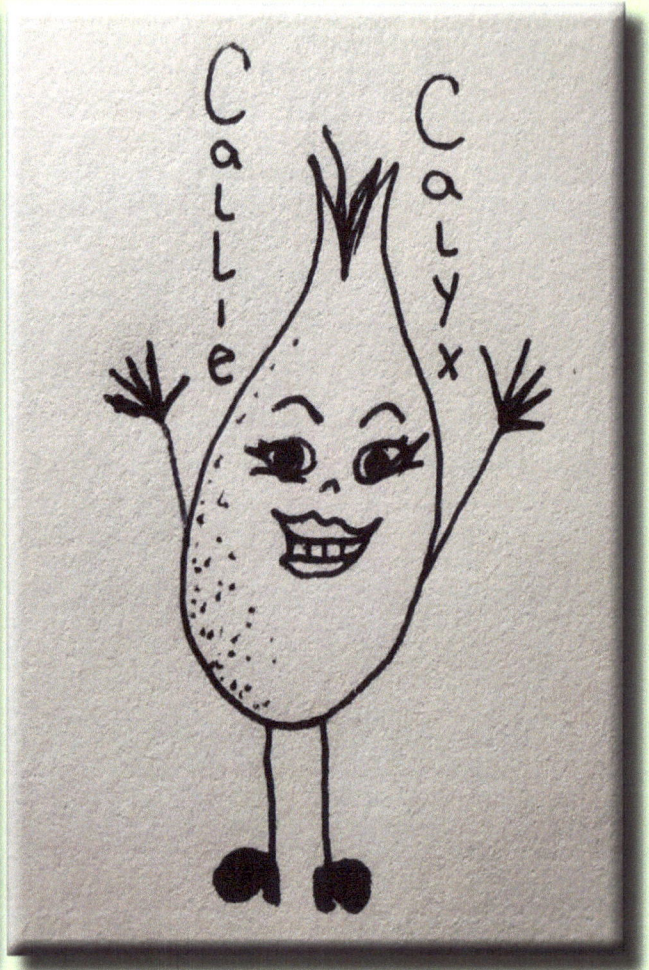

Callie Calyx

This is Callie, she is a Calyx. Her job is to protect the buds so they can bloom into flowers. The flowers are what most people look for to use for help. Callie is a very important part of the plant as well, without her who knows what might happen to our next friend!

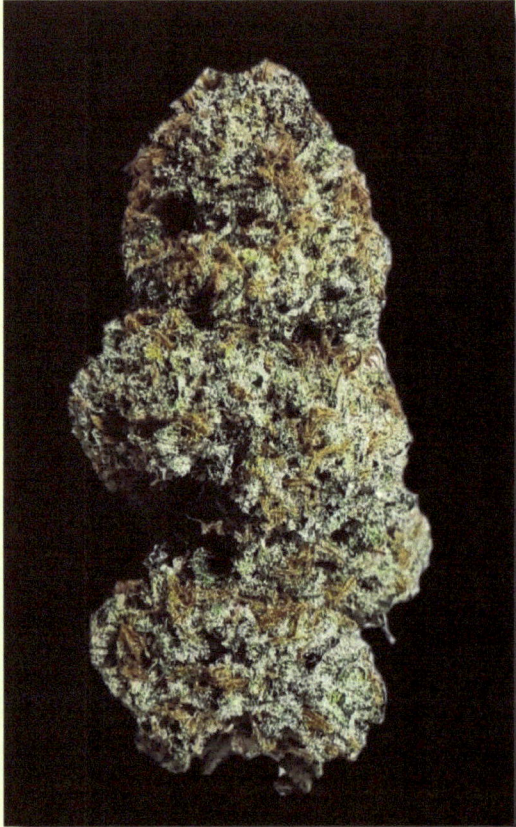

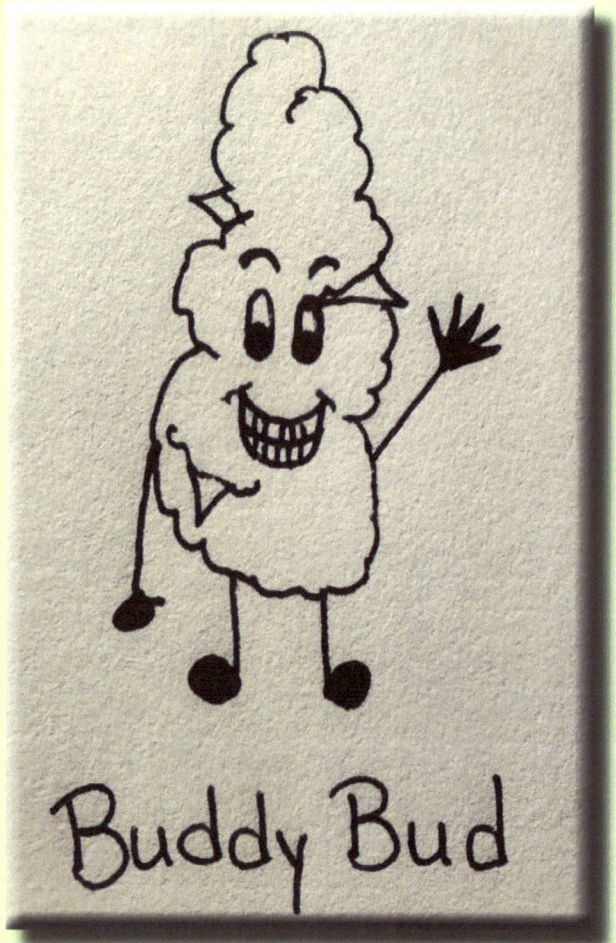

Buddy Bud

Buddy Bud

This is who Callie has to protect! Meet Buddy Bud. He is the bud who blossoms into a beautiful flower to be consumed by patients who use cannabis as medicine. He holds most, if not all, of the smells and flavors!

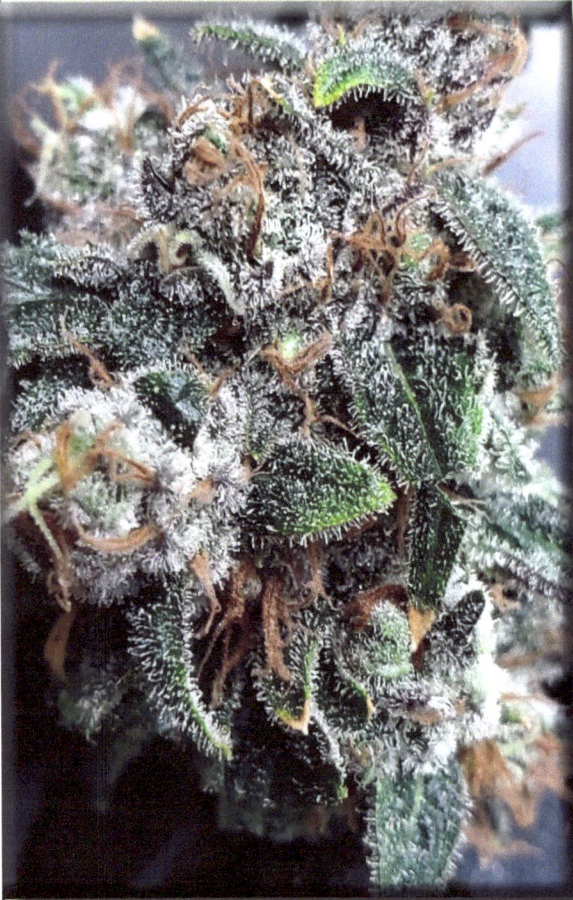

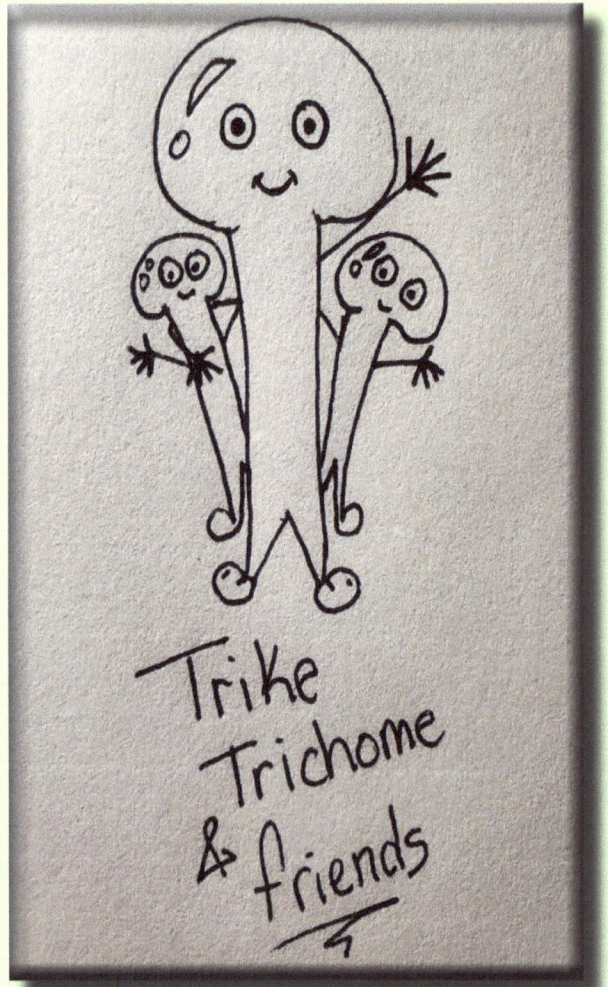

Trike
Trichome
& friends

Trike & Friends

Trike is a Trichome. He and his friends hold all the terpenes and THC in their pockets. Trichomes are <u>translucent</u> mushroom shaped crystals that are attached to the buds/flowers. They make the flowers look sparkly! See how pretty they are?

Did You Know?

There are multiple types of this plant?

- Ruderalis
- Industrial Hemp
- Sativa
- Indica
- Hybrid

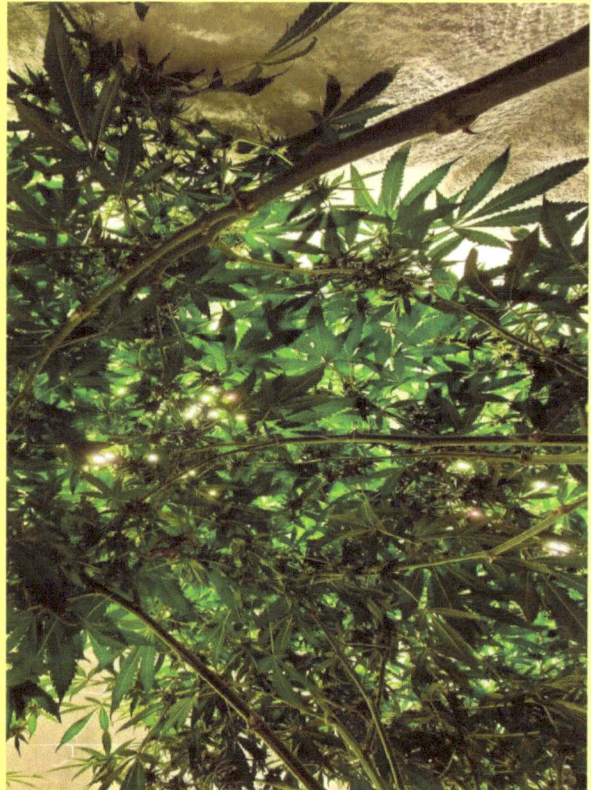

Did You Know?

- RUDERALIS IS A TYPE OF CANNABIS PLANT THAT ONLY HAS 5 LEAVES AND DOESN'T HAVE MUCH <u>MEDICINAL</u> VALUE

- SATIVA PLANTS HAVE LONG, SKINNY LEAVES AND LIKE TO GROW TALL.

- INDICA HAS WIDER LEAVES AND IS USUALLY QUITE BUSHY.

BOTH INDICA & SATIVA CAN HAVE +/- 9 LEAVES

Industrial Hemp

Usually grown on a large scale for goods, hemp has very low THC level and is used for creating Hemp-<u>Derived</u> CBD products. Hemp is better suited for use as fuel, paper, building materials, etc. Did you know, using more hemp products could possibly save the planet?

Indica vs. Sativa

According to early research Indica <u>strains</u> have a more relaxing effect and make people want to sit back and enjoy a movie or read a book. Sativa is said to have the opposite effect, giving you

energy and more focus and motivation. Some people even feel the opposite reactions.

Fun Facts!

- Cannabis plants can get sick if not properly cared for, just like humans
- Some bugs are great to keep around, like the praying mantis and lady bugs!
- Some strains are determined to live and can grow anywhere with hardly any help
- There are boys and girls just like us! The boys make pollen which cause the girls to produce seeds in their flowers
- Cannabis plants can grow well into the double digits is well cared for!
- Did you know that these plants use nitrogen, and that if you have rainwater and it storms that your rainwater becomes charged with nitrogen?
- Did you know that the cannabis plant needs rest? Yes! They sleep too!

Definitions

- <u>BLOOM-</u> To produce flowers; be in flower

- <u>HERB-</u> Any plant with leaves, seeds, or flowers used for
flavoring, food, medicine, or perfume.

- <u>HARVEST-</u> the process or period of gathering in crops.

- <u>PSYCHOACTIVE-</u> Affecting the mind

- <u>NON-PSYCHOACTIVE-</u> Not producing an effect (such as changes in perception or behavior) on the mind or mental
processes

- <u>TRANSLUCENT-</u> (of a substance) allowing light, but not
detailed shapes, to pass through;

Definitions

- <u>DERIVED</u> – obtain something from (a specified source).

- <u>MEDICINAL</u> – (Of a substance or plant) having healing properties.

- <u>STRAIN</u> – a breed, stock, or variety of an animal or plant developed by breeding.

- <u>NUTRIENT</u> – a substance that provides nourishment essential for growth and the maintenance of life.

- <u>CBD</u> – Non-Psychoactive Cannabinoid found in the cannabis plant, Cannabidiol

- <u>THC</u> – Psychoactive Cannabinoid found in the cannabis plant, Tetrahydrocannabi-nol

- <u>CANNABINOID</u> – any of a group of closely related compounds which include can-nabinol and the active constituents of cannabis

- <u>GERMINATE</u> – (of a seed or spore) begin to grow and put out shoots after a period of dormancy

www.ingramcontent.com/pod-product-compliance
Lightning Source LLC
Chambersburg PA
CBHW041551040426
42447CB00002B/138